THE REVOLUTION IN MEDICINE

THE REVOLUTION IN MEDICINE

BEING THE SEVENTH HAHNEMANNIAN ORATION DELIVERED OCTOBER 5TH, 1886, AT THE LONDON HOMOEOPATHIC HOSPITAL

BY

JOHN H. CLARKE, M.D.,

GYAN

Published by

Gyan Publishing House
5, Ansari Road
Daryaganj, New Delhi-110002
Phone: 011-47034999, 9811692060
E-mail: books@gyanbooks.com

Distribution Network
gyanbooks.com
India, USA, Canada, UK, Australia, France

ISBN : 978-81-212-6595-9 (PB)
First Published, 1886

2nd Impression 2022

Printed at: Gyan Press, Delhi.

THE REVOLUTION IN MEDICINE
Author: JOHN H. CLARKE

THE

REVOLUTION IN MEDICINE.

BEING THE SEVENTH HAHNEMANNIAN ORATION DELIVERED OCTOBER 5TH, 1886, AT THE LONDON HOMŒOPATHIC HOSPITAL.

BY

JOHN H. CLARKE, M.D.,

Physician to the London Homœopathic Hospital; Lecturer on Materia Medica to the L.H.H. Medical School.

1886.

THE

REVOLUTION IN MEDICINE.

CONTENTS:

I.—DARKNESS AND DAWN.

NIGHT.

1786.

HAHNEMANN.

A REFORMER NOT A DESTROYER.

IN THE VALLEY OF THE SHADOW.

DAWN.

I.—DARKNESS AND DAWN.

NIGHT.

LADIES AND GENTLEMEN,

One hundred years ago the Art of Medicine still lay wrapped in Cimmerian night. The power of the Dark Ages, which the Protestant revolution had rolled away two hundred years before from other pursuits and avocations of men, unfettering the intellect in science and the conscience in the moral world, still lingered like a trailing, inky cloud after a storm over all that concerned the treatment of sick humanity. No ray of reason pierced the impenetrable fog of theory and conjecture in which the ministers of Healing moved, blindly led by blind Tradition, and blindly worshipping the fetich, Authority. Now and again the bolder spirits had ventured, like Paracelsus, to rise in revolt against the ruling powers of darkness; but in their attempts to break the rusted and corroding chains of Authority—chains, which to the generality were a glory instead of a shame—they had succeeded in breaking only themselves. Systems of treatment based on fanciful theories of disease had risen, had had their day, and had sunk into their native night. Discoveries in anatomy and physiology has been made—and had left the practice of medicine no better than before. A century and a half had passed since Harvey wrote the treatise which contained his grand induction of the circulation of the blood —an induction, be it here remarked, honestly made from anatomical observations, and not, as is commonly alleged, from the observation of vivisected animals,—thus completing the work of Servetus, Realdus and Cesalpinus, who had been before him in the field and had paved his way. But Harvey did not dream of saying a word against the prevalent custom of bleeding for almost every disease—or, indeed, of suggesting any improvement in the Healing Art. So absolutely without effect on practice had Harvey's great discovery proved to be, that in the succeeding generation the physician in ordinary to the son of Harvey's master, the second Charles, published a work* on "mummiall quintessences," among which a quintescence to be distilled "in the month of June or July" out of a "great quantity of overgrown old toads" was one the least objectionable.

1786.

In the year of our Lord, 1786, when the Old Régime in France was rapidly approaching its tragic end, and when the man who was destined to master the wild forces of the impending revolution, and to lead them through the length and

* *Aurora Chymica*, by Edward Bolnest, M.D., Physician in Ordinary to King Charles II.

breadth of Europe, overturning thrones and dynasties and shaking to their foundation the social and political institutions of the western world, was a young lieutenant of Artillery in his nineteenth year,—in this year a man who was born to inaugurate a very different revolution—to put an end to the reign of Darkness in the world of Medicine,—already twelve years the great soldier's senior, was a general medical practitioner in the town of Dresden, dreaming as little as the other of the great part in the world's history he was to be called upon to play.

At this date Hahnemann was innocent of homœopathy.

HAHNEMANN.

I must not trench too much on the ground so ably occupied by my predecessors in this place, who have spoken of Hahnemann, the Man and the Physician, Hahnemann as a Medical Philosopher, as the Founder of Scientific Therapeutics, and of Hahnemann and his Works; but it will not be possible for me to avoid it altogether. And though some of the ground may be old, the recent publication in English of the great work by the lamented Dr. Ameke, of Berlin, *Homœopathy: its Origin and its Conflicts*, translated by Dr. Drysdale, of Cannes, and edited by Dr. Dudgeon, opens up much that is both valuable and new.

Who, it may be asked, was Hahnemann, that he should set himself to revolutionise the most conservative of arts, the profession in which the worship of ancestors was observed with a piety more than Chinese?

Samuel Hahnemann was the eldest of a family of ten born to a painter on porcelain, of Meissen, in Saxony. His father, whose means were none too ample, destined the boy to follow the same trade as himself. But when God has special work for a man in this world He does not leave his upbringing entirely in the hands of his parents. As a child Hahnemann shewed an intense passion and a wonderful aptitude for learning. When his father removed him from school (as he did for long periods together), with the aid of a clay lamp of his own construction the child continued his studies in his chamber at night after the less congenial labours of the day. But his teachers would not part with such a scholar without making great efforts to retain him. At last they prevailed on the father to allow the boy—whose health had given way under the combined effects of hard manual labour and chagrin—to follow his bent, they offering to forego all fees for his instruction. Such was the confidence he inspired that when only in his twelfth year Herr Müller, the principal of the Meissen School—of whom Hahnemann always speaks with the greatest veneration and affection,—commissioned him to teach to others the elements of Greek. At the age of twenty he removed to Leipzig to begin the study of medicine, his last school essay being entitled "The Wonderful Construction of the Human Hand." As showing his appreciation of his father's treatment of him, much as he had been thwarted and opposed, a note of Hahnemann's, written years afterwards, may be quoted here :—

"In Easter, 1775, my father sent me to Leipzig, with the sum of twenty thalers —the last money that I ever received from him. He had to bring up several children on his limited income, and this sufficiently excuses the best of fathers."*

Thus the struggle with adverse circumstances began in Hahnemann's

* Ameke, p. 151.

childhood; and there can be no doubt that this early lesson in enduring hardness formed one of the most important elements in the training for his after life. At Leipzig the struggle continued. Hahnemann supported himself by teaching and by translating for publishers whilst he diligently attended the medical classes of the University. Here his fees were remitted by virtue of a kind of Government foundation instituted for the benefit of poor and deserving students. After two years spent at Leipzig he removed to Vienna in order to study medicine practically, since Leipzig possessed no hospital. At Vienna he attended the Hospital of the Brothers of Charity, in the Leopoldstadt, under Quarin, the Physician in Ordinary to the Emperor. Like most of his preceptors, Quarin conceived a great liking for the young Hahnemann, for whom he showed his partiality by taking him with him on his visits to private patients. "He singled me out," says Hahnemann, "loved and taught me as if I were his sole pupil in Vienna, and even more than that, and all without expecting any remuneration from me." * To the genuine teacher a pupil of Hahnemann's kind is himself a sufficient reward. It is to Quarin's lasting honour that he discovered Hahnemann's worth; and the love and the care he bestowed on his pupil were seeds sown in a fertile soil. A post of resident physician and library custodian to the Governor of

* Ameke, p. 152.

Transylvania, obtained at Quarin's recommendation, enabled Hahnemann to replenish his scanty resources, and at the same time to pursue his practice and his studies. In 1779 he took his M.D. degree at Erlangen, where the graduation fee was lower than at Leipzig; thence he returned to his home, and after a short residence at Dessau removed to Gommern in 1781. Two years later he married Henrietta Küchler who shared with him for nearly fifty years the storms, the labours and the trials of his life. He now removed to Dresden, where we have already seen him, and where he remained for about six years practising his profession as best he might, and making good use of the electoral library.

A REFORMER NOT A DESTROYER.

If a man would inaugurate a new and better era in any department of human affairs, it is first of all necessary that he should master what there is of good in the old. He comes not to destroy but to fulfil. So Hahnemann, long before he commenced the work by which he is now almost exclusively known, had made himself in all the branches of his Art, and even in those which are now regarded as subsidiary branches, not merely proficient, but one of the first authorities of his time. Chemistry at this day owes to Hahnemann's genius, among other things, the discovery of the best test for metals in solution; and the apothecaries, who were destined to be the first to cast the legal stone at him, possessed in his *Pharmaceutical Dictionary*—a work of immense labour, learning and research, which took him years to complete,—their most valuable and most indispensable friend. His early writings prove him to have been far in advance of the men of his day. The practices of "fashionable physicians" he freely criticised; and in place of their violent measures he praised the virtues of cold water and fresh air in a way that would surprise modern sanitarians who imagine that hygiene is a discovery of the latter half of the nineteenth century. His learning in all that concerned his Art was unrivalled. No writer of eminence, living or dead, escaped his wide reading and scholarship, whilst his wonderful memory retained for his use almost everything that he read.

IN THE VALLEY OF THE SHADOW.

But before Hahnemann was ready to enter on the external conflict he must first feel the power of the Darkness in his own soul and conquer it there. In spite of his great powers and high intelligence,—nay, rather by very reason of them—the seemingly never-ending night of Medicine oppressed him to the dust. Where smaller and less sensitive natures could live and move without discomfort a Hahnemann could not breathe. At last he could bear it no longer; he had reached, he thought, the "Everlasting No" of Medicine, and he gave up the practice in despair. Removing from Dresden in 1789, he came again to Leipzig, and there supported himself and his family by working as a literary hack, enduring the hardships of extreme poverty rather than continue to kill his fellow-creatures—as he felt he was doing — in accordance with the rules of his art. But illness in his own family recalled him to himself. He felt, as he believed in the goodness of God, that there must be a real Healing Art, if only it could be found.

DAWN.

This was the darkest hour before the dawn. Just then Hahnemann was engaged in translating Cullen's work on Materia Medica from English into German; and when he came to that part of the work which deals with Peruvian Bark, he was dissatisfied with the attempt Cullen made to explain the curative action of the drug in ague. It occurred to Hahnemann that if he were to try the effect of the drug on himself in health, he might obtain some information as to its action in disease. He therefore took an ordinary dose of the powdered bark. Within a short time he was seized with an attack of chills and fever indistinguishable from a fit of ague. Thinking this might possibly be a genuine attack of ague and not the result of the dose, after a little delay, he repeated the experiment, and again the same result followed. He had now no longer any doubt; and the exactness of his observation has since been confirmed by numberless similar experiences. Bark cured ague: and bark could also cause the very counterpart of ague in the healthy. This was the first ray of light which heralded the coming dawn. Further experiments on himself with bark and other drugs proved that this was no isolated experience, but an instance of a general rule: that there was a definite relation between the action of a drug on the healthy and its action on the sick, and that by knowing the one the other might with certainty be predicted.

With the breaking in of light upon his own mind Hahnemann was restored to hope and life.

But unlike certain modern discoverers who are eager to rush before the public with every idea that comes into their minds lest another should come before them and claim the priority (which is really not worth the claiming), Hahnemann took care to make sure his ground before he made any definite announcement. His translation of Cullen was published in 1790. For six long years he worked at the subject before he published his famous Essay "*On a New Principle for ascertaining the Curative Properties of Drugs*," in which the homœopathic principle was first clearly made known to the world. The essay was published in the leading medical periodical of the day, *Hufeland's Journal*, and it bears to the practice of medicine much the same relation that Harvey's essay on the *Motion of the Heart* bears to physiology. The essay excited much comment at the time of its appearance, as it was bound to do, but no one suspected it then of being heretical, whilst its great originality and power were acknowledged on all hands. It was not until he had laboured still three-and-twenty years in developing his system, had collected around him an enthusiastic band of disciples, and had won the confidence of a large circle of patients, that his medical brethren—and especially the apothecaries — became alive to the dangerous nature of his teachings and practice, and put in operation against him the favourite engine of the Dark Ages—persecution.

The new light which had dawned in this way upon Hahnemann's mind shed its rays before and after; illuminating and explaining much of the experience of the past, as well as indicating the path by which advance was to be made in the future. In numbers of the cases of cure recorded in ancient writings, as Hahnemann shewed, the drugs which had been given had removed conditions the like of which they were capable of causing when administered to those in health.

In his *Essay on a New Principle* Hahnemann formulates his conclusion thus :—

" *Every powerful medicinal substance produces in the human body a peculiar kind of disease, the more powerful the medicine, the more peculiar, marked and violent the disease.*"

"*We should imitate nature* which sometimes cures a chronic disease by superadding another, and employ in the (especially chronic) *disease we wish to cure, that medicine which is able to produce another very similar artificial disease, and the former will be cured; similia similibus.*"

This proposition has never been shaken. Denied it has frequently been; misrepresented it still is; disproved it cannot be.

Hahnemann had now his foot upon the solid ground of fact. The weakness of all previous systems of treatment that had been proposed lay in their having been founded on the quicksands of theory. If Hahnemann had first sought to find some supposed explanation of the fact made plain to him, and if he had then sought to build up a system upon the explanation instead of upon the fact, his system would have fared no better than the others. Facts are durable things; explanations are always changing.

On his own body Hahnemann "proved" a large number of drugs; that is to say, he took them in substantial doses when in health and observed the effects that followed. These he noted as they occurred and made no attempt to explain them, simply labelling them what they were, "positive effects." Drugs, like human beings are apt to be at times a little inconsistent in their actions. For instance, belladonna will cause some persons to perspire profusely, and will make the skin of other persons dry. Like a sensible man, Hahnemann, instead of trying to reconcile these inconsistencies, or to find an ingenious explanation of them, preferring, as smaller men are wont to do, his own explanation to the facts, simply set down both as "positive effects." An observer of the old school seeing one of these effects would immediately dub the medicine a "sudorific," and another seeing the opposite effect would be equally certain to dub it "anti-sudorific;" and each would go away satisfied that he possessed a scientific understanding of the drug's action, and for ever after use it according to the name he had given it, ignoring as exceptional all contradictory experiences. So it has been; and so it is to this day among those who reject Hahnemann; and hence the confusion that prevails in the works of orthodox writers on Materia Medica, to the distraction of the unhappy student who is compelled to learn their contents — for examination. Hahnemann swept away all these delusive names, embodying at the best only partial experiences, and suffered the much abused drug to write out its own character in the symptoms and changes it produced in his healthy body; he performing the simple clerical duty of writing, so to speak, to the drug's dictation. By so doing, Hahnemann has made it possible for us to know the actual powers, the very characters in fact, of hundreds of substances now in daily use in homœopathic—and allopathic !—practice.

At the time when his essay was published Hahnemann was a physician of the highest standing and repute (which no one then thought of questioning), and in the forty-second year of his age. A physician who knows nothing but drugs is, properly speaking, no physician at all; but a physician who does not know how to use drugs is a man without his right hand. Hahnemann was no one-sided enthusiast—he was an accomplished physician in all other matters apart from his knowledge of drugs and his skill in the use of them; and he was thus in every way qualified to lead the reform in the most important of all the divisions of the Doctor's Art — the treatment of the sick by drugs. For the question of drug-action barred the way of all progress; and so long as the practice of drug administration remained unreformed, so long as the absurd theories and the high-sounding, delusive terms in which they were embodied held dominion over the physicians' minds, the inauguration of a better era was impossible. But now that the light had come to him, Hahnemann was fully equipped and ready to enter on his life's great work, for which all before had been a preparation. He was not alone in bewailing the state of the practice of his time, nor was he alone in his discernment of the curative powers of drugs; others, like Von Stoerk, had possessed an insight of a limited kind into the properties of drugs, and saw the necessity of giving them singly, before Hahnemann. But there was none who saw a way out of the darkness until he came; there was none who was able to gather up the good and shew how it might be recognised and distinguished from the mass of the bad. He alone possessed the genius, the talent, the learning, the faith and the fortitude that were needed to withstand all the powers arrayed against him, to lead all those who would follow him into a region of light, and to compel all those who refused to follow, to cease at least to do evil, if they would not learn to do well.

II.—THE THREE-FOLD WORK.

CLEANSING THE AUGEAN STABLE.

CONSTRUCTIVE AND DEFENSIVE.

UNEXPECTED ALLIES.

II.—THE THREE-FOLD WORK.

CLEANSING THE AUGEAN STABLE.

Hahnemann's work was of a three-fold kind. He had first to clear his ground of the rubbish of ages, taking care to preserve everything of value that lay concealed among the heaps; he had to build a new edifice on the ground he cleared; and all the time he had to defend his work and himself against the attacks of his numberless foes, the blind lovers of darkness, the pharisaic sticklers for the old order, right or wrong. For, as there were those in the days of Plato who would rather be in error with him than be right with any less authority; and, as, in Harvey's time, almost all his professional brethren declared that they would rather be wrong with Galen than be "circulators" with Harvey; so at the beginning of this boasted Nineteenth Century of ours—and I fear not at the beginning alone—the medical profession were almost unanimous in preferring to slay with Galen *secundum artem*—according to the most approved rules of their art—than to heal with the revolutionary Hahnemann. And verily they did slay *secundum artem*, as we shall presently see.

The one measure most relied on by the physicians of Hahnemann's time in their endeavours to combat disease was blood-letting. Next in importance to this came the administration of complex mixtures, the prescriptions for which were regarded as in themselves works of art to be compiled as carefully as a sonnet, almost as much for the admiration of awe-struck apothecaries as for any possible good the compounds might do to the patients. Hahnemann's keen eye soon perceived the folly and the wrong of both of these fashionable measures. In 1791,* just when the idea of homœopathy had taken possession of his mind, we find him writing of blistering and bleeding in this philosophical strain:—"It is the common

* Translation of "Monro's Materia Medica," Vol. II., p. 275. Ameke, p. 76.

delusion that the sores produced by vesicating agents only remove the morbid fluids. When we consider that the mass of the blood during its circulation is of uniform composition throughout, that the exhalents of the blood-vessels give off no great variety of matter under otherwise identical conditions; no rational physiologist will be able to conceive how a vesicating agent can select, collect and remove only the injurious part of the humours. In fact the blister under the plaster is only filled with a part of the common blood when it is drawn from a vein. But according to the insane idea of these short-sighted doctors, venesection, too, draws off the bad blood only, and continued purging only evacuates the depraved humours. It is terrible to contemplate the mischief which these universally held foolish ideas have caused."

In the following year, 1792, Hahnemann's sentiments on this question brought him for the first time into open conflict with his professional brethren. He alone of all men had the courage to criticise publicly the medical treatment of the Emperor Leopold II. of Austria, who died *secundum artem*, in this way.—

"The monarch was on the 28th of February attacked with Rheumatic Fever"—This is the report of Lagusius, the Physician in Ordinary to the Emperor, with a running commentary (in the brackets) by Hahnemann;—"and a chest affection [which of the numerous chest affections, very few of which are able to stand bleeding? Let us note that he does not say pleurisy, which he would have done to excuse the copious venesections if he had been convinced that it was this affection.] and we immediately tried to mitigate the violence of the malady by bleeding and other needful remedies [Germany—Europe—has a right to ask: which?]. On the 29th the fever increased [after the bleeding! and yet] three more venesections were effected, whereupon some [other reports say distinctly—*no*] improvement followed, but the ensuing night was very restless and weakened the monarch [just think! it was the night and not the four bleedings which so weakened the monarch, and Herr Lagusius was able to assert this positively], who on the 1st of March began to vomit with violent retching and threw up all he took [nevertheless his doctors left him, so that no one was present at his death, and indeed, after this, one of them pronounced him out of danger]. At 3.30 in the afternoon he expired, while vomiting, in the presence of the Empress."*

Commenting on the case elsewhere Hahnemann said: "His physician, Lagusius, observed high fever and swelling of the abdomen early on February 28th; he combated the malady by venesection, and as this produced no amelioration, three more venesections were performed without relief. Science must ask why a

* Ameke, pp. 88, 89.

second venesection was ordered when the first had produced no amelioration. How could he order a third ; and, good Heavens ! how a fourth, when there had been no amelioration after the preceding ones ? How could he tap the vital fluid four times in twenty-four hours, always without relief, from a debilitated man who had been worn out by anxiety of mind and long continued diarrhœa ? Science is aghast ! "*

But bleeding was not to be abolished at one blow. Hahnemann strove against the practice with all his might, and for years the neglect of bleeding continued to be the chief sin of homœopathy in the eyes and mouths of its opponents. But except in the practice of Hahne-

* Ameke, p. 88.

mann and his followers bleeding continued to be the favourite method of treatment; and it was only when the immeasurably and incontestably superior statistics of homœopathic over the ordinary treatment emboldened some practitioners of the unreformed faith to leave their patients without any medical treatment at all that they began to perceive the truth of Hahnemann's teaching—that bleeding was slaying. When they left their patients to Nature their death-rate fell in an amazing way, though it still remained distinctly higher than that of homœopathists. It is now the fashion to ascribe the discontinuance of blood-letting to certain experiments on animals performed by Marshall Hall. This is a very pretty story, and quite good enough for those who wish to believe anything rather than the truth of their indebtedness to Hahnemann; but the wise know well that great reforms are not brought about in that way. Another ingenious device for robbing Hahnemann of his credit due is the theory advanced by some that diseases have changed their type since his time, and that the Sangrado bleeders of the past were quite right in their bleedings, and that Hahnemann was quite wrong in denouncing them. This is another pretty story; but the race of blood-letters is not yet entirely extinct, and the results the modern Sangrados have to show bear a striking resemblance to those of their fore-runners, notwithstanding the supposed "change of type" in disease.

Witness the case of Count Cavour. On May 29th, 1861, Cavour was taken ill, in the midst of his parliamentary duties, with chills, followed, after some hours, by pains in the bowels and vomiting. He was bled the same night, and again the next day both morning and evening. On the 1st of June he was again twice bled. On the 2nd of June the wound in the arm re-opened during an effort, and further bleeding took place. On his doctors attempting to bleed him again (this time at the request of Cavour himself, who thought that nothing else could relieve him of his sufferings, which were really the result of the bleedings he had already been subjected to) no blood would flow. Quinine was then given. Cavour asked that it might be given in pills, instead of in solution, because he knew from experience that the solution would make him vomit. The doctors would not consent to this, and violent sickness ensued. The next day he was cupped and blistered, but the blisters could not be made to rise. King Victor Emmanuel, who visited the minister, proposed to his doctors that they should open a vein in his neck. This proposal they were about to take into consideration, when they were saved further trouble by the death of the patient. Cavour died suffering from unquenchable thirst.* It may fairly be said that Cavour resisted the treatment he received better than the Emperor Leopold, although the illness

* Ameke, p. 261.

of the latter occurred before the supposed "change of type" of disease had been discovered. The proposal of Victor Emmanuel to still further deplete the already bloodless man met with a singular nemesis when some years later, within the memory of us all, he himself perished—*secundum artem*—of his sanguinary doctors.

These historic examples will serve to show how firmly rooted in the medical mind was the idea that blood-letting was a necessary thing, and how much courage it demanded on Hahnemann's part to depart from the received tradition. His attitude on this question caused him to be denounced as a murderer—for denying his patients the "benefits" of blood-letting!—throughout the medical world, and cost him the friendship of some of the ablest physicians of the day who had previously been on terms of the closest intimacy with him.

Hahnemann early emancipated himself from the dominion of the complex prescription: but it cost even him a severe struggle. It was considered then the highest mark of proficiency to combine a large number of ingredients in the same prescription, arranging them artistically under the imposing names of *basis* or principal, *adjuvans*, *corrigens*, *dirigens* and the rest,—which were supposed to "assist," "correct" and "direct" the action of the ingredient in chief. When Hahnemann had the courage to prescribe only one thing at a time, he could not help feeling a little ashamed of the mean opinion the apothecaries were sure to form of him, the apothecaries who made up the prescriptions being paid in proportion to their length. The opinion of the apothecaries with regard to Hahnemann did not improve with time.

In 1797, the year following that in which his epoch-making "Essay on a New Principle" was published, Hahnemann contributed another notable paper to *Hufeland's Journal*, entitled, *Are the Obstacles to Certainty and Simplicity in Practical Medicine insurmountable?* In this article he delivers himself as follows:—

"Who knows whether the *adjuvans* or the *corrigens* may not act as *basis* in the complex prescription, or whether the *excipiens* does not give an entirely different action to the whole? Does the chief ingredient, if it be the right one, require an *adjuvans?* does not the idea that it requires assistance reflect severely on its suitability, or should a *dirigens* also be necessary? I thought I would complete the motley list, and thereby satisfy the requirements of the schools.

. . . .

"The more complex our prescriptions are the darker is the condition of therapeutics . . . How can we complain of the obscurity of our art when we ourselves render it obscure and intricate?"*

* Ameke p. 78.

In the same year in which he first publicly attacked blood-letting, 1792, Hahnemann shewed his courage in departing from the evil traditions of his profession in another matter of great importance. In his day, and long after his day, it was the custom to treat lunatics as if they had been wild beasts. Hahnemann protested against the wickedness of this practice, and his cure of the Hanoverian Chancellor Klockenbring by gentle means is a matter of European history. "I never allow an insane person," says Hahnemann, "to be punished either by blows or any other kind of corporal chastisement, because there is no punishment where there is no responsibility, and because these sufferers deserve only pity and are always rendered worse by such rough treatment and never improved."* After his complete cure, Klockenbring, "often with tears in his eyes," shewed Hahnemann "the marks of the blows and stripes his former keepers had employed to keep him in order."*

Thus Hahnemann anticipated another of the improvements in medical practice fondly imagined to be a discovery of recent years and credited to Englishmen. All honour to the English doctors for the work they did, and the reform they brought about; but the originality is not theirs—it belongs to Hahnemann.

* Ameke, p. 67.

CONSTRUCTIVE AND DEFENSIVE.

Hahnemann did not spend all his powers in fighting the abuses of his time. All the while, he was assiduously working out his idea, testing the action of medicines on his own healthy body, and building up his system on the solid ground of his observed results. In the year, 1810, he had so far perfected his system that he was able to publish his celebrated *Organon*, in which he set forth in detail what he had briefly sketched in his *Essay on a New Principle*, fourteen years before. In the following year he applied to the University of Leipzig for permission to teach medicine under its authority. The Senate of the University were not very well disposed to entertain his request, but they said that if he would write a thesis, and defend it before them, his request should be granted. Hahnemann readily complied, sending in his *Helleborism of the Ancients*, a work of such extreme merit that his censors could not find in it a single fault, and granted him the licence to teach forthwith. For eight years he continued thus to teach and to practise, aided now by an enthusiastic band of disciples, and supported by a large section of the public. But there was a growing feeling of jealousy among his professional brethren, and the apothecaries came to like him less and less. For Hahnemann had discovered that besides the great advantage there was in giving only one drug at a time—a very grave sin of itself in an apothecary's eye—there was no need to give a poisonous dose of even that one drug in order to obtain its curative effects. This was altogether too much for the equanimity of the apothecaries. Their craft was in danger. One medicine at a time, and not much of that!—how was a poor apothecary to live? On the principle of securing the greatest good to the greatest number—apothecaries being many and Hahnemann only one—they determined to extinguish Hahnemann. There was a law in Germany forbidding a physician to make up his own prescriptions. This proved an admirable opportunity for the boycotting proclivities of the trade. They refused in a body to dispense any prescription of Hahnemann's, and when he dispensed his own medicines, even though he made no charge for them, they put the law in force against him, and so procured his banishment from Leipzig in the year, 1819. He was then in the sixty-fifth year of his age. After long and painful wanderings from state to state, he at last found an asylum in the little town of Coethen, under the egis of the friendly Duke of Anhalt.

UNEXPECTED ALLIES.

When Hahnemann went into exile he left behind him enthusiastic disciples to carry on his work and develop his system. Hahnemann might be exiled, but homœopathy was not extinguished. And homœopathy had allies little reckoned on by its foes. Epidemics in their courses fought for homœopathy. Contagious fevers which swept off the patients of the old school doctors spared those of Hahnemann and his followers. Perhaps the most potent ally homœopathy has ever possessed has been the dreaded cholera. It is often said that homœopathy is all very well for children, and for mild diseases in adults; but no stretch of allopathic ingenuity can make of cholera a mild disease, or a disease peculiar to children. Yet it remains on the testimony of their own witnesses—allopathic doctors appointed under Government authority and prejudiced against the system of Hahnemann—that wherever homœopathy and allopathy have been tried in epidemics of cholera side by side, the results of the homœopathic treatment have proved immeasurably superior to those of the allopathic. This is a fact which it remains for our opponents to explain; they cannot explain it away.

Hahnemann, ere he left Leipsig, had already made his work's foundation sure, and had rendered impregnable the house of his fame. Thirty-three years had passed over his head since we first found him at Dresden. The storm of the French revolution had burst and had passed. Napoleon had had his day and had fallen from his high estate. Amidst all the political turmoil of his time, and the storms of his own life, Hahnemann had accomplished a work which was destined to bring about a rèvolution fraught with the happiest consequences not to Europe only, but to the whole civilised world.

III.—THE REVOLUTION AND THE MAN.

1785 AND 1886.

MEDICAL DOGBERRYS.

THE MAN.

III.—THE REVOLUTION AND THE MAN.

1786 AND 1886.

Let us now come to our own day and compare the darkness of 1786 with the comparative light of 1886. In the sixteen years and upwards during which I have been connected with the medical profession as student or practitioner I have never once seen a patient bled. In all truly civilized countries bleeding now occupies the very last instead of the first place among the means of cure. The habit of prescribing a number of drugs in the same mixture is not yet by any means extinct, especially in country districts; but the practice of giving one drug at a time is rapidly gaining in favour even among allopathists, and no one now dreams of skilfully building up a prescription of *basis*, *excipient* and the rest, as in itself a work of art. The leaders of the allopathic section are approaching the "Everlasting No" of prescribing,— the point Hahnemann reached in 1789—for they openly declare that they have little or no faith in drugs; and when one of them succeeds a homœopathist in the care of a case of acute disease he thinks the best thing he can do is to give the patient no medicine at all. The effect of the Revolution in Medicine, of the deliverance from the tyranny of the Dark Ages, has been felt in every home in christendom. The lancet, the leech, and the fearful concoction are no longer the haunting terror they once were from the cradle to the grave. Douglas Jerrold's death-bed appeal to the doctor who insisted on cupping him—"Why torture a dying creature, doctor?" has been answered by Hahnemann—Why indeed?

An abler pen than mine has sketched the debt of the children to "The great Deliverer."—

"Children," says Miss Cobbe, "noticing the busts of Hahnemann in the shop windows, may be properly taught to bless that great Deliverer who banished from the nursery those huge and hateful mugs of misery—black founts of so many infantine tears—mugs of sobs and sighs and gasps and struggles unutterable, from one of which Madame Roland drew the first inspiration of that martyr spirit which led her onward to the guillotine, when she suffered herself to be whipped six times running, sooner than swallow the abominable contents."* The influence of Hahnemann is everywhere. It presses like an enveloping atmosphere, and, like an atmosphere, so insensibly that it may be unperceived. We find it in the home; in the hospital; we find it in allopathic books. It may be denied; and even by those who have consciously helped themselves to his works

* *Sacrificial Medicine*, in *The Peak in Darien*, by Frances Power Cobbe, p. 196.

it may be ignored; but it is there, and history will not fail to declare it.

MEDICAL DOGBERRYS.

I know it is the fashion to say that the improvement must have come with the growing enlightenment of the age; but the answer to the simple-minded persons who make this statement—and who remind me of worthy Dogberry, when he said, "to read and write comes by nature,"—the answer to them is, that with all the growing enlightenment of the previous centuries, the improvement did not come, and until Hahnemann pointed out the way no one had any notion how medicine was to escape from the darkness of erroneous theories, and the chains of dead Authority. It was only by the immeasurably superior results of Hahnemann's treatment over their own that the opposing section were, "at long and last," as the Scotch folk say, induced to give up their barbarous practices, and to leave the sick man at least a chance of getting well. Those who like may believe in the wonderful effects of Marshall Hall's vivisections: the deliverance of Medicine from bondage was wrought by the heroic struggles of Hahnemann for light, begun in his childhood, and carried on during long years of privation, of labour and of persecutions, and maintained with a fortitude rarely seen among the sons of men, and never seen except when founded, as Hahnemann's was, on a mighty faith in the goodness of God, and in his own commission. This is the kind of thing, and this only, which can bring about such a beneficent Revolution as this century has witnessed in Medicine: and since the world is not altogether under the dominion of evil, a career like that of Hahnemann can never be wasted or lost.

THE MAN.

Such was Hahnemann, and such was his work. The discovery that he was an ignorant charlatan is one of the many remarkable allopathic discoveries — not to say inventions — of the last half century. In his own day his works were too well known to admit of such slanders gaining credence. Base motives and his criminal neglect of blood-letting were the chief stones thrown at him then. But Hahnemann was not to be destroyed by persecution, and he was too great a man to make any querulous complaint of that which he endured. "I care nothing," he says, in 1828, "for the ingratitude and persecutions which have pursued me on my wearisome pilgrimage; the great objects I have pursued have prevented my life from being joyless."* And on his death-bed, when it was remarked that Providence owed exemption from suffering to him who had already suffered so much in his efforts to relieve others, he replied with all his old fire, "Why should I expect exemption from

* Chronic Diseases, I. 8. Ameke, p. 163.

suffering? Every one in this world works according to the gifts and powers which he has received from Providence, and *more* or *less* are words used only before the judgment-seat of man, not before that of Providence. Providence owes me nothing. I owe it much. Yea, everything."†

That Hahnemann had faults and failings I do not deny, any more than I deny that there are spots on the face of the sun. But we do not refuse to own that the sun warms us and gives us light because we have discovered the spots; and to see them at all we require to look through darkened glass. There

† Ameke, p. 167.

may be some persons dim-sighted enough to see the spots—and even to see spots where there is none—without such help, and foolish enough to deny that the sun shines. Such, it seems to me, are those mentally purblind persons who see so plainly the defects (real or imagined) in Hahnemann's character that they cannot bring their magnanimity to allow him any credit at all.

Some there are who cannot see a hero, even when placed fairly before their eyes. Their insect range of vision is so narrow and so low that they see nothing clearly that is much greater than themselves; and their minds are so much in subjection to their eyes that they will not believe in anything they cannot see. But these are not the men to measure Hahnemann. His fame lives not in their breath. His fame has firm foundations; it is sure as the everlasting hills. It may be hidden from little minds by the little reputations of to-day, as the snowy peak of some sky-piercing giant may be hidden from view by hillocks close at hand; but as, when distance levels meaner heights, the monarch of the range towers over all the scene, so as years roll on will the name and fame of Hahnemann tower over the plains of history, when the little reputations of to-day shall have mingled indistinguishably with the common dust.

IV.—OUR INHERITANCE.

THE REVOLUTION NOT COMPLETE.
"MEDICAL ETHICS."
EN AVANT!

IV.—OUR INHERITANCE.

THE REVOLUTION NOT COMPLETE.

But great as the work of Hahnemann is, and great as is the Revolution he has brought about, the Revolution is not yet complete. It is true, there are in the United States of North America upwards of 10,000 practitioners of medicine following in the footsteps of Hahnemann, and all the world over the positive—as well as the negative—benefits of the new method are known. It is true, also, that allopathic professors, after filling their books with the records of their labours in torturing dumb brutes, and endeavouring in vain to extract from these some therapeutic pabulum wherewith to allay the cravings of their famishing pupils, are fain to present them with a dish of crumbs furtively swept from Hahnemann's floor. But this by no means contents us. As Hahnemann's heirs, much remains for us to accomplish. He has shown us the better way; it is for us to go forward. We must develop our inheritance, and defend it against the attacks, overt and covert, of those in power in the profession. We must make our case plain to the people, who are the ultimate judges and masters of either medical school.

"MEDICAL ETHICS."

There is much talk in these days about Medical Ethics. In the minds of our opponents Medical Ethics is an invention of recent date, expressly or mainly designed for the purpose of putting down homœopathy. Ladies and gentlemen, the only principle of medical ethics I know, is the good of the people; and for each individual doctor the people are represented, first and foremost, by his individual patients; and after that, according to his powers, by the world at large. The profession exists for the people. But this is scarcely the view of the allopathic section. In this country strong men—yes; even strong Scotchmen!—dare not do the thing they own to be right, because, forsooth! their College says they must not: and this is what they understand by medical ethics. Over the Atlantic, in the Land of Freedom, the same "code of medical ethics" holds sway; and because some have ventured to rebel against the old commandment of the Dark Ages of Medicine, "Thou shalt extinguish the light,"—which is, being interpreted into the language of to-day, "Thou shalt boycott homœopathy,"—fierce civil war has broken out in the allopathic ranks.

EN AVANT!

So long as this state of things continues—so long as the allopathic materia medica remains the most hated and hateful of the studies of the medical curriculum; so long as its professors present their students with the torturings of dumb creatures as the only source of progress in the art of prescribing, and slander Hahnemann whilst they steal homœopathy, and for the most part mar what they steal; so long as the student is hindered from following the dictates of his own conscience by the pressure of authority and professional opprobrium;—so long must we be at work and in arms. There is a comfortable maxim of which we are all very fond, "Truth is great and will prevail." Yes; but also—lies are great, and at present *they* prevail; and unless we walk in Hahnemann's steps, and endeavour with all our might to set forth the truth as it should be set forth, lies will prevail to the end. Truth is worth working for and fighting for; and truth demands it. We may sit at home cozily repeating our beautiful maxim, like the American editor in the time of the war, who could not fight—much as he liked fighting—because he had to remain at home to announce from day to day the inspiriting news that "the Government were about to take vigorous measures to put down the rebellion;" but if we all do this, the liberation of medicine will never be complete—the lies will prevail to the end. The same strenuous efforts, the same faith and fortitude which enabled Hahnemann to accomplish all he did, are demanded of us, according to our measure, to maintain what he began. We lament that our powers are so small, and our numbers so few; we wish with all our hearts that the great men opposed to us (and their greatness we do not call in question) would bring their great powers to work the rich field which is altogether too vast for us to overtake, instead of using the weight of their names to resist our efforts and to dissuade those who would from following in the better way. Still we are not discouraged; we are doing what we can. Our little hospital here stands out as a witness for the truth, and though we could wish that it were larger, and our own skill more worthy, we have no reason to be ashamed of the position it holds among the institutions of the metropolis. Its wards are open for the inspection of those who wish to learn; and for those who have time to attend regular classes provision is made for systematic teaching in the School of Medicine with which the hospital is combined.

We are doing what we can; and we hope to do yet more in the time to come. The Revolution is progressing. But the progress is slow; and those who hate knowledge are many. Our work is for Truth and Justice and Light. To all who love Justice and are not afraid of Truth we look for help in our endeavour to break down what still remains of the tyranny of Darkness in Medicine, and to hasten the coming of the perfect Day of Liberty and Light.

THE END.